# THE BELLY FAT DIET BOOK

## Why the Flat Belly Diet is The Ultimate Plan for Melting Belly Fat

# By Mackenzie Jagger

*http://theflatbellysolution.org*

# Other Books
# By
# Mackenzie Jagger

Mackenzie Jagger

## The Paleolithic Diet
### What It Is and Why It Works

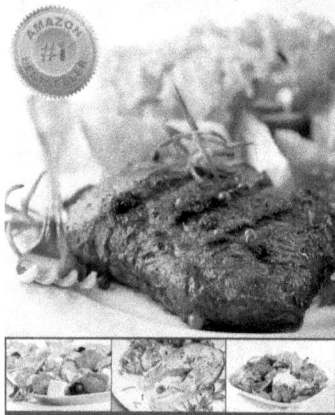

This book is dedicated to all those who have struggled to eat healthily and maintain a modest weight.

May this book be a new beginning for you!

**To Your Success!**

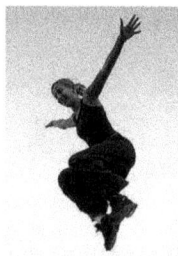

# Table of Contents

# INTRODUCTION

Hi, this is Mackenzie Jagger.

What you'll find in this book is the exact information you need to know to succeed with the Flat Belly Diet.

If you're like me, there are times when you just don't want to read over 350 pages to ascertain the essence of the material. In today's fast paced society many of us feel that less is more, which is why I decided to extract the most important information I found inside "The Flat Belly Diet" written by Liz Viccariello and Cynthia Sass.

In 2008 the editors of Prevention magazine took the world by storm when their Best Selling book explained that the number one body part most people would like to change could actually be targeted! They discovered an unknown key to fighting belly fat, now backed by science that anyone can take advantage of.

Please note! If you are looking for the most comprehensive Belly Fat Diet Book, I recommend the original Flat Belly Diet by Liz Viccariello and Cynthia Sass. That is the book that this book is based on.

I made this book short (and succinct) for a reason: I want you to get started quickly, to take away every excuse you have for not losing your belly fat and put a smile on your face when you start to see the results!

This is a 32 day diet but the knowledge you will gain regarding how and what to eat will stay with you for a lifetime.

\*\*\*\*\*

Here are a few of the things you'll learn in this book:

- Why belly fat is worse than other fat that you would have on other parts of your body?

- What are MUFA's and what are their 5 categories?

- What are the 3 Rules of the flat belly diet?

- Discover why the authors say that the diet is about "food and attitude"

- Why the Flat Belly Diet is The Ultimate Plan for Melting Belly Fat

# **Chapter One**

## Insuring Optimal Success with the Flat Belly Diet

Individuals experience weight gain for a number of reasons throughout their lives, and outside of wanting to look good for the people around you, there are numerous personal reasons why you should want to lose weight, including personal appreciation, and maintaining proper health. Weight gain can occur with age, medical conditions including depression and diabetes, or lifestyle changes including pregnancy, surgeries or career changes. Life can catch all of us off guard, changing our routines at a moment's notice, which in return can alter our eating habits until the next thing you know we are avoiding an entire section of our closets as a result.

Weight gain delivers a blow to your self-esteem, your personal energy level, and compromises your ability to feel great about the clothes you are wearing. The larger problem becomes that once you put the weight on, especially around the abdomen, it can be extremely difficult to shed. Diet and exercise can help you lose weight, but if you have been down that road before, with little results, it becomes increasingly difficult to want to try again. Unlike regular dieting options, the flat belly diet can help you lose that stubborn stomach pouch, and keep it off. With a combination of focus, determination, exercise and increased diligence when it comes to exactly what you are putting inside your body, you too can have the flat stomach that you have always wished for in just over a month.

# Chapter Two

## What is the Flat Belly Diet?

The flat belly diet is a very specific weight loss plan that targets stubborn belly fat, and helps burn your fat's existence by as much as seven pounds in the first 96 hours of use, equaling an amazing loss of five inches around the waist in as little as four days. Overall, with continued use and understanding of the program, dieters can lose 15 pounds in a little over 30 days with this structured dieting program. Although the diet targets mostly women who are 40 and over, it is an acceptable and proven method for belly fat reduction in men and women of all ages.

The flat belly diet concentrates on stomach fat because although all extra weight creates an unhealthy existence, stomach fat is exceptionally unhealthy, and can lead to greater difficulties later, including decreased physical activity, high blood pressure, diabetes, heart disease, sleep apnea, stroke and degenerative diseases. Belly fat can become increasingly dangerous as it multiplies over time, and can result in visceral fat that stores itself around important bodily organs, creating an insulin resistance. Part of the science of the flat belly diet is to lower insulin levels through the consumption of monounsaturated fat, which also increases triglycerides, both of which aid in weight loss.

Consuming a diet high in monounsaturated fats allows you to target the stubborn belly fat directly, without giving up all of the foods you love. Essentially, the diet allows you to eat specific foods while losing weight, without the use of exercise.

Although the plan is very specific, and its success level is through the roof, the first week of the program can be incredibly challenging, especially to those who are new to dieting. It is important to keep a positive outlook, while staying focused and aware that once you are through the first week, the results will speak for themselves. After the hard part is over, you will be ready to proceed with the balance of the diet while looking forward to maintaining its scientific approach to weight loss to receive the maximum results.

The main focus of the diet is to consume four, 400 calorie meals every four hours of each day, which includes an approved, healthy snack in the morning or afternoon. Each of these meals should include a monounsaturated fat enriched food, which will be outlined below in the food options section of the book to help you gather meal ideas that provide the most success.

## What are Monounsaturated Fats?

Monounsaturated fats, also called MUFAs, are healthy fats that have been scientifically proven to reduce stomach fat. The advantages of consuming meals that contain these fats aren't simply their ability to zap belly fat, but the fact that they consist of some of the most delicious and satisfying foods available.

Avocados, nuts, seeds, oils, olives and even dark chocolate fall into the MUFA category, which means you can eat some of your favorite foods while undergoing a physical metamorphosis at the same time.

# Chapter Three

## Flat Belly Diet Meal Plans

Consuming four, 400 calorie meals each day will require planning and foresight, which in turn requires a dedicated commitment to the diet, prior to beginning the first week's stringent plan.

Although the meal preparation itself is not time consuming, you will want to plan your trips to the grocery carefully, insuring you have the approved foods available at all times, so you can mix and match their preparation as you see fit, without straying from the program to consume more convenient, but less healthy options, in your cupboards.

Meal plans can include delicious options such as breakfast tacos, egg & cheese sandwiches, turkey wraps, hummus, baked chicken & vegetables, and even peanut butter cookies! The diet revolves around eating lean cuts of fish and chicken, with measured fruit and vegetable options that are easier to eyeball for serving sizes than they are to weigh, so do not be discouraged by the use of measurements in any of the food examples that exist throughout the book. A good rule of thumb in this instance is to measure your servings by the size of your fist, if you do not have a measuring cup on hand.

*The First Week: Put on Your Game Face!*

The first four days of the program are considered a "Jumpstart" to the process, which will alleviate the overall bloated stomach symptoms that you live with every day – whether you know it or not – while preparing the digestive system for a new diet plan that will help erase belly fat quickly and effectively. This portion of the diet is incredibly important to its success, so be sure that you are able to commit to the overall process before you begin. The restrictions are tough at first, but once you get through this week, you will be able to introduce a bunch of your favorite foods into the mix, so hang in there and stay positive!

There are several main points to the Jumpstart program, which will help your success rate including:

- Training Your Brain to Eat Slowly:

Take small bites, and chew your food completely

• Eat four, 400 calorie meals each day that follow the plan EXACTLY

• Enjoy a Five Minute Walk after Each Meal

• Drink Two Liters of "Sassy" Water Each Day

## The First Four Days of Meal Plans

Before we get into the actual food options, there are a number of things you need to avoid during the first four days of the diet, so start clearing out your cabinets to avoid the temptations!

**Salt:** Salt and water combine in your system and create excessive bloating, which is exactly what the first four days of the diet is trying to reduce. Consuming salt, which can include simply using the salt shaker, or certain seasonings (check the labels for the sodium content that is included in some of your favorites, but obviously "seasoning salt" is out), can cause excessive bloating.

**Processed Foods:** Processed foods are chock full of preservatives, which is a fancy use of sodium. Stay away from anything unnatural, including packaged foods.

**Carbs:** Reduce your carb intake by cutting out breads, pastas and potatoes for the first week of the diet. These items take longer to digest, and are counterproductive to the first week's goals of diminishing excess bloating.

**Gas Inducing Vegetables:** Say goodbye to broccoli, cabbage and onions during the first week, to avoid bloating. These gas-heavy vegetables and legumes such as beans and lentils can be reintroduced later in small servings.

**Sugar Substitutes:** If it comes in a packet, or lists itself as low-calorie, under the guise of acting as a sugar, skip it completely.

**Coffee, Tea & Hot Chocolate:** Since you cannot shake your favorite sweetener into your morning coffee, it should provide you with a good reason to skip it altogether. These drinks are high in acid, and can upset the cleansing process.

**Alcohol, Carbonated Drinks & Fruit Juices:** Again, high acid intake can disrupt the process and place an unwanted strain on the GI tract while it is being prepped as your new diet plan. Stay away from these excessively bloating liquids altogether.

**Fried & Spicy Foods:** Fried foods are

always a terrible idea, but especially during your first week of the flat belly diet. Spicy foods, although they can be delicious, and a great departure from the same types of meals day in and day out, operate like fried foods in your system, digesting slowly, causing increased bloating.

## What is "Sassy" Water?

Sassy water is named after one of the diet's creators, and can be concocted with the following ingredients, which can help you decrease bloating, while settling the GI tract to prepare it for a healthier diet.

You will need a large pitcher, which you will consume the contents of each day, so be sure and make the container as accessible as possible, maybe purchasing one with an airtight lid, or something easy to transport to the office or gym. Some find it helpful to make an entire pitcher, and divide the contents into reusable water bottles, so they are accessible at home, work, during workouts, in meetings or in the car.

The following ingredients must sit overnight once combined, so plan ahead for each of the four days, so you are never without this important component of the diet. We typically make a new batch before we go to bed, so when you awake the next morning, we are ready to go!

## Combine into One Pitcher:

• Two Liters of Water, Which Equals Approximately 8.5 Total Cups

• One Teaspoon of Freshly Grated Ginger

(Peel the ginger, and grate it with the small section of cheese grater directly into the container, atop the water)

• One Medium Cucumber, Peeled and Sliced into Thin Rounds

• One Medium Lemon, Sliced into Thin Rounds

• Twelve Whole Spearmint Leaves

# Chapter Four

## Appropriate Diet Structure
## & Food Options:

### Days One through Four

During the first four days of the program, you will need to be incredibly stringent about your diet, to enjoy the optimal benefits. Here is how your meals should be structured for the first four days. The great news about this diet is, if you are one of those people who skip breakfast, or eat on haphazard occasions, like when you have time, instead of at scheduled times throughout the day, or even if you're one of those people who do not eat at all on some days, this program will help train your body to eat at beneficial times, allowing you to enjoy a much healthier lifestyle in the long run.

## Breakfast Diet Structure

- One Dairy Product
- One Starch Product
- One Fruit
- Seeds
- Water

### Appropriate Breakfast Food Options

- One Cup, Skim Milk
- One Cup Corn Flakes or Rice Krispies (alternate option: any puffed wheat cereal)
- One Half Cup of Pineapple
- One Quarter Cup of Sunflower Seeds
- One Glass of Sassy Water

### Lunch Diet Structure

- One Dairy
- One Protein

- One Vegetable
- Water

### Appropriate Lunch Food Options
- One Serving of Light String Cheese
- Three Ounces of Chunk Light Tuna, in Water (always avoid the oily version)
- One Cup of Carrots
- One Glass of Sassy Water

## Snack Diet Structure & Option
- One Fruit Smoothie: Contents should include One cup of fat-free yogurt, and one half cup of fruit.

## Dinner Diet Structure
- One Vegetable
- One Protein
- One Starch
- Olive Oil
- Water

## Appropriate Dinner Food Options

• One Cup of Mushrooms, Sautéed in One Teaspoon of Olive Oil

• Three Ounce Chicken Breast, Grilled or Baked

• One Half Cup of Steamed Brown Rice

• One Glass of Sassy Water

These items can be mixed and matched, but should always follow the same structure for each of the four days. The menu will widen as the diet develops, so the program will become easier as time goes on. Be sure to drink the entire two liters of Sassy water each day, as it is as important to the diet as the foods you consume.

*****

# Chapter Five

## Flat Belly Diet Exercise Program

One of the most appealing parts of the flat belly diet is that exercising is not necessary to achieve the expected results. However, it is beneficial to keep in mind that physical activity is the cornerstone of a healthy body. Combining a healthy diet with regular exercise can help you achieve your weight loss goals exponentially. Even if you do not have time to hit the gym every day, there are a number of activities you can participate in, without going out of your way!

## Take the Stairs

If you work in an office that is on the third floor, or even better, the eighth floor, start skipping the elevator each time you arrive or depart and take the stairs. Depending on which floor your office is on, you can start out slowly by skipping the elevator once a week, adding another day as you feel comfortable, as you so not hurt yourself with the increased activity. This practice will help maximize your workout opportunities in the office, and will land you at your desk feeling rejuvenated.

## Run Errands on Foot

Even if you are simply grabbing a smoothie in the middle of the day, walk to the yogurt shop, instead of getting into your car and driving. If you need to go to the bank, or drop by the post office, walk to both if they are within a reasonable distance from your home or office. This will not only give you a break from your business day, but also help extend your physical activity for the day.

## Park Farther Away

Although there are very few things more rewarding than finding a premier parking spot, the benefits of parking so close to the entrance are even less rewarding. Look for a parking spot as soon as you pull into the parking lot of any local retailer, shopping mall or grocery store, and walk the remaining distance to the entrance, to maximize your physical activity.

# Start Saying Yes!

When friends, family or coworkers ask you to join in a game of volleyball, softball, kickball or even tag with the kids, say yes, get up and enjoy the fun! Not only will you be interacting socially, but you will be exerting physical energy that will help you lose weight in the long run.

Once you have increased your physical movement throughout the day, consider extending that activity by taking a bike ride or going hiking on the weekends. Exercise does not have to take place in a gym, or with an instructor present, it simply has to consist of physical movement, and can easily become something you enjoy, instead of something you dread. If you need motivation, consider asking friends or coworkers to join you on walks around the office at lunchtime or around your neighborhood in the evenings. It really is that simple!

Now let's move forward with the plan and start talking about the actual diet, and food options. Once you are finished with your four day jumpstart, things will start looking brighter, and more relaxed. You will still need to remain disciplined and focused, but there are a lot more meal alternatives for you to enjoy now that you have made it through the first week, which should increase your optimism.

# Chapter Six

## Regular Menu Options

### *Breakfast*

Instead of only puffed grains, you can introduce oatmeal or an English muffin into your diet in the mornings, which will allow you to feel fuller until your next meal. One cup of apple almond oatmeal or a toasted, whole-grain English muffin with peanut butter (two tablespoons only!) are both excellent choices. Another great option is granola and fat-free vanilla yogurt. Simply measure one cup of fat-free yogurt into a bowl, and pile one half cup of strawberries or blueberries atop the vanilla flavored treat and enjoy!

More fun, and flavorful breakfast options include...

## Waffles Florentine

Toast two whole grain waffles, and top them with two tablespoons of black olive tapenade, one scrambled egg white (cooked in spray, not butter), and one half cup of spinach. Serve alongside one half cup of grapes.

## Spanish Eggs

Separate one egg white into frying pan using a teaspoon of olive oil. Add an additional, whole egg atop the egg white and fry both sunny side up for flair, or flip it to your heart's content! Place the cooked eggs on top of a six inch, whole wheat tortilla (this can be warmed in the microwave, if you would like), and layer one half cup of salsa and ten large, sliced green olives on top. You can roll it up burrito style, or eat all of the ingredients separately!

## Almond Butter Toast with Fruit

Toast one slice of whole grain bread in the toaster and smear two tablespoons of almond butter atop it while it is still warm. Pair the delicious, buttery treat with one half cup each of strawberries and kiwi.

## Lunch

Lunch items should focus on lean cuts of chicken or fish, paired with salads, fruits and avocados. You can use this combination in any form, as long as you use it smartly. Avoid large buns, or processed breads when making sandwiches, and think more along the lines of pita bread or whole-grain English muffins. Adding pesto and tapenades to sandwiches gives them a great kick, and provides a fresh alternative to the less healthy condiment options including mayonnaise.

Here are a couple of examples...

## Salmon, Avocado & Grapefruit Salad

Combine three cups of romaine lettuce with two ounces of canned, wild salmon (store the rest for another day's luncheon), one quarter of an avocado and a whole grapefruit (this can be eaten separately, but a peeled and parted version adds to the sweetness of the dish, providing a nice contrast to the fish and avocado). Top the salad with one tablespoon of rice vinegar, and two teaspoons of olive oil.

## Ham (Turkey or Chicken), Cheese & Pesto Sandwich

Spread one tablespoon of pesto over a whole-grain English muffin and add your favorite lean cold cut in the form of ham, turkey or chicken, taking care to only use one serving. Add one slice of the low-fat cheese of your choice, and layer lettuce and tomato on top for a complete and robust meal. Couple the sandwich with a vegetable in the form of carrots or grape tomatoes and you will have a complete, healthy meal.

## Roast Beef Deli-style Sandwich

Pile three ounces of lean, deli roast beef on one slice of whole wheat bread, and add two tablespoons of green olive tapenade to the second piece of bread before closing the sandwich to enjoy. For a twist from the same old deli style, toast the bread before preparing the sandwich to add warmth to the meal. Slice a whole, medium sized pear in half, and enjoy the treat!

## Sensational Chicken Lettuce Wraps

Divide a standard head of Bibb lettuce into leaves, until you have six total. Divide two tablespoons of hummus evenly between the leaves before dividing three ounces of grilled chicken atop the hummus smeared leaves. Distribute two tablespoons of walnuts over the opened leaves, roll and eat! Partner this delicious meal with one cup of raspberries and you will feel energized in no time!

## Super Summer Salad

When vegetables are fresh, you can enjoy a beautiful salad tossed with pine nuts, as many times of the week as you would like! Simply slice two tomatoes and placed them atop one cup of arugula leaves. Add two ounces of sliced, part-skim mozzarella cheese, five slices of red onion and douse with two tablespoons of pine nuts, and one teaspoon of olive oil. For an extra zest, shake a few dashes of balsamic vinegar atop the whole concoction, while delivering a pinch of pepper to taste. Skip the salt. You won't need it!

## Waldorf Salad in a Pita Pocket

Load one whole wheat pita pocket with two, light garlic and herb (or flavor of your choice) cheese wedges, one medium apple, chopped; two tablespoons of walnuts, and one cup of shredded romaine lettuce.

# Mediterranean Salad

Toss chickpeas, cherry tomatoes (halved or whole), one cucumber (chopped or sliced), and ten large black olives into a bowl with one tablespoon of lemon juice, and serve with toasted, whole wheat pita slices.

## Dinner

Dinner is the perfect opportunity to introduce starch into your meals, giving you the options of steamed brown rice, which comes in ready to eat, single serving containers now-a-days, so all you have to do is microwave them, or whole wheat pastas, which like its brown rice counterpart in a box, can be prepared ahead of time, so your meals are ready when you are. In fact, preparing your meal's staples at the beginning of the week will help keep you regimented and on course to succeed, so it is always a good idea to plan your shopping trips around the week's meals, and prepare them so you always have the appropriate foods ready. If you have had a long day at the office, you may not want to go home and cook, which can lead to you side-stepping the diet. If your meals are prepared, you simply have to warm them up when you get home, and start relaxing immediately following. Some delicious and exciting dinner meal examples are listed below. Keep in mind, lean cuts of fish and chicken are going to be your staples for the next month, so get excited about how you mix and match them.

## Grilled Salmon & Vegetable

Grille one, three ounce salmon steak and pair it with one and one half cup of steamed green beans and two tablespoons of almonds.

## Salmon & Snow Pea Pasta

Combine one cup of cooked whole grain spaghetti style pasta with one tablespoon of extra virgin olive oil, one teaspoon of minced garlic, one quarter cup of canned salmon (drained and rinsed), and one half cup of snow peas. Toss the concoction fully to deliver the maximum flavor from all of the ingredients.

## Tuna, Pepper & Olive Pasta Salad

Combine one half cup of cooked, whole wheat pasta spirals with one pouch or can (in water) of chunk light tuna, two tablespoons of light balsamic vinaigrette, one quarter cup of diced green (red or yellow) pepper, and ten large black olives, sliced. Toss the combined ingredients in a single bowl, and refrigerate until cold. This is a perfect meal to prepare in the morning, so when you return from the office, your dinner is served directly out of the refrigerator.

## Snacks

It is important to understand that snacking is imperative to this diet. Whether your cravings come in the mornings or in the middle of the afternoon, you should satiate them with a healthy, flat belly diet approved snacking option, to help keep your diet on track. Too many times, for reasons no more exhausting than pure convenience, diets are thrown by the wayside in favor of preservative-filled vending machine snacks. Not only are they unhealthy, but they are loaded with sugar, sodium and fat. How else can they survive inside of that device so long? Steer clear of these diet-killers, and plan accordingly by incorporating any of the following snacks into your shopping trips, and having them on hand at all times.

## Hummus, Pine Nuts & Red Peppers

This is our favorite, because the combination is delicious, and it is incredibly filling, so we are able to make it through the afternoon reenergized, and quite full.

Spoon one quarter cup of hummus onto a plate or bowl, and sprinkle two tablespoons of pine nuts over it (you can eat these separately, if you would like). Scoop the dip with one cup of red, yellow or green pepper strips and enjoy the incredible taste combination it creates.

# Fruit, Veggies, Cheese & Crackers

Enjoy one four ounce can of pineapples in juice, one cup of baby carrots, and six, small whole wheat crackers with one serving of light string cheese at your desk in the afternoon, to hold off any cravings until dinnertime. Add two tablespoons of peanuts to the mix, and your appetite should be completely satisfied.

# Apples & Popcorn

Another great snacking option is to cut one medium sized apple into wedges, and top it with two tablespoons of peanut butter. Pair the fruit portion of the snack with four cups of light, trans-fat free microwave popcorn, and you will have solved any salty and sweet cravings for the day.

No matter how you plan to lose weight, even with a plan as simple as the flat belly diet, it will not take long to become discouraged, or to feel uneasy about your progress. This happens with all diets, workouts and new activities so do not allow yourself to feel overwhelmed. If you need to repeat the initial four days again, you certainly can. This diet should work at your pace, so if you are traveling excessively, or under a lot of stress, and either of the two disrupted your first attempt at the flat belly diet, try again. The benefits of losing excess belly fat are immense, and can be categorized in two separate segments: Health & Appearance.

Keep in mind, once you get the hang of healthy options, they will be easier to add to your meals. Think in terms of light cheeses and lean cuts of meat. Avoid sauces, or anything you would normally "pour" onto your foods for flavoring. Buy crunchy, colorful vegetables, and keep them handy at the office and at home, so you are less likely to sabotage your diet. Thinking ahead and being prepared are two key components of successful dieting, because the moment you have to step outside of your healthy routine, you are going to feel the effects. Those effects could be in the form of you beating yourself up about it later, which you shouldn't do, since every diet is interrupted at some point, or in the form of not feeling well because of the preservatives you packed away during a moment of weakness.

Once you are eating healthier, your body will begin to crave the attention and fresh foods you have begun feeding it, so take advantage of it! Find the things in the Flat Belly Diet that you like, especially at first, so you do not feel overwhelmed by the process. If you have to eat the same few things every couple of days, so be it!

Certainly variety is the spice of life, but getting you on track to a healthier existence is more important at first, so think in terms of what you already like. This approach will make life so much easier for you, and you will still benefit from the success at the same time.

## A Note for Vegetarians & Vegans

Anyone can participate in the Flat Belly Diet, but it is important to note that some of the key components of the diet's success are the adaptation of protein. Since protein typically comes from animal sources, whether they are meat, fish or poultry, it could be harder for a vegetarian to work around the diet's approach. However, there are a number of vegetables, nuts and seeds that will provide protein without the involvement of meat. Likewise, eggs and cheeses can comprise a significant source of protein for those of you who do not eat meat, so take advantage of the offerings as they fit into your diet. The menus provided in this book are simply suggestions to give Flat Belly Dieters the direction they need to live healthier lives. If there is something in the menu that does not suit your personal, vegetarian diet, skip it. You are free to work around the ingredients so they cater to your tastes and lifestyle. Again, the idea is to start eating things you like that are good for you, not change your lifestyle choices.

With that said, if this diet appears challenging to a vegetarian, there is a pretty good chance that it is going to seem downright impossible to a vegan. However, both the vegetarian and vegan can benefit from the use of tofu substitutes where the recipes call for a meat or protein source. Likewise, where eggs and cheese are listed as ingredients, use the vegetarian or vegan substitutes that are available at your local market. Take care to check the labels to insure the sodium content isn't extreme, and follow the balance of the diet accordingly with things you can eat, including delicious fruits, vegetables, oatmeal and even pancakes!

Keep in mind that the importance of this diet's success, and the meal recommendations that encompass it, revolve around the addition of monounsaturated fats, or the MUFAs identified earlier in the book. These items, avocados, nuts, seeds, oils, olives, all fall into the vegetarian and vegan approved diets, and can be added to any meal effortlessly.

Here are a couple of sensational menu options for either herbivore group...

# Fresh Veggie & Basil Wrap

Decide on a wrap that suits you, whether it is whole wheat, tomato, spinach or red pepper (there are so many delicious and exciting options available, it is a wonder anyone eats bread anymore!), and spread it with two wedges of light cheese spread of your choice (Laughing Cow works beautifully, and the garlic and herb option is to die for!). For the vegan, substitute the cheese with two tablespoons of hummus. Add one quarter cup of avocado, one sliced tomato, a selection of fresh basil leaves and finish with one teaspoon of balsamic vinegar.

## Avocado & Mango Delight

Try a delicious and colorful salsa option that will have you buying mangos by the cartload! Peel and cube one whole mango, and place it in a bowl. Add one quarter cup of diced avocado, two tablespoons of cilantro, and finish the mix with the juice from half of a lime. Sprinkle the delightfully fresh mixture with cracked black pepper, or even crushed red pepper to spice it up a bit. Serve the dish with one large tortilla, toasted and cut into wedges.

## Veggie Burger Deluxe

Add one, fully cooked black bean veggie burger to a whole wheat bun before placing one cup of mixed baby greens, one quarter cup of canned corn, and one quarter cup of sliced avocado to the patty. Douse two tablespoons of salsa over the sandwich before adding the top of the bun, and enjoy this deluxe sandwich with a southwest flair!

# Sesame Slaw Salad

Mix two cups of broccoli slaw with one quarter cup of red pepper slices, one quarter cup of canned water chestnuts, one orange – cut into pieces – into a bowl. Sprinkle two tablespoons of sesame seeds over the mix, adding two tablespoons of rice vinegar and one tablespoon of sesame oil to the salad. Mix the contents completely, and refrigerate until cold.

These simple recipes are not simply for vegetarians and vegans. They can be added to any dieter's menu options and enjoyed any time of day or night. It is important to concentrate on adding the MUFAs to each meal segment, instead of focusing on the contents of the meal. As long as it is less than 400 calories, and you are enjoying these meals four times a day, you will begin shedding that stubborn belly fat in no time.

Don't forget to treat yourself with dark chocolate from time to time, just so you do not forget that you deserve to eat the finer food groups of this diet as well! Also, do not forget about trail mixes that contain nuts and dark chocolate, as a snacking option. Just be sure to abide by serving sizes listed, skipping the salted versions, and to insure that your entire day's intake doesn't consist of the delicacy. Although trail mixes are perfect for office snacking, you do not want to skip a more balanced meal as a result of the convenience.

When you are shopping for food items, always search for things that are fresh, and that suit your lifestyle. Trying to change too much about yourself too quickly could result in failure. Think about all of the diets you have tried before, and get ready to take hold of the new you with the Flat Belly Diet. The ease exists, you just have to work within the parameters, and start enjoying life as the new, thinner you!

*****

# Chapter Seven

## The Benefits of the Flat Belly Diet

Toting around excess belly fat can lead to several things, including a lowered self-esteem, ill-fitting clothing and an unhealthy body. Maintaining the flat belly diet for 32 days can transform your body and mind into a proactive, happy and good looking version of your old self.

## *Health Benefits*

Belly fat can hide deep within the body, so even those who have no outward appearance of belly fat can still be affected by its internal existence, which is called visceral fat. This fat hides deep within the stomach, taking refuge around important organs and tissues that your body needs to operate at an optimum level. When the fat takes hold of these areas, it requires the body to work harder in an effort to complete its normal, involuntary functions. This stress can lead to high blood pressure, diabetes, and stroke. The flat belly diet helps cleanse these areas of their hostage taking fats, allowing your body to work optimally, with less exertion, which means you will be healthier in the long run.

## *Increased Energy*

It is no secret that when you lose weight you are able to move with more agility, as you become more willing to participate socially in physical activities. Whether you are simply taking up co-workers on their offer to walk at lunch, or are joining in a club softball league, losing weight helps you feel better, giving you a sense of inclusion. And with the increased energy levels you will continue to burn more calories and fat, toning more than just your stomach in the process.

## *Appearance*

Fitting into an outfit that you haven't worn in a very long time increases your self-esteem ten-fold. Not only are you feeling better, but you look fantastic, which will not go unnoticed by those around you. Smaller sized clothes could mean a shopping excursion for great reasons this time around, instead of buying a bigger size, which could send anyone into a depressed state. Enjoy the new you, and show off your new body with a great outfit that complements your commitment to working hard to lose weight.

## *Attitude*

Now that you are able to control your appetite cravings, and have physically seen and felt the benefits of the diet, you will take on a new, positive approach to situations and life in general. Conquering a diet plan provides a tremendous amount of accomplishment to the psyche, and you deserve every bit of praise you receive from others, and yourself. Be proud of your success, and share your knowledge with others in an attempt to spread good cheer and exciting, healthy opportunities for those around you. You now have the look and health you have always wanted, so why not boost both attributes with a healthy, shiny attitude towards life as well?

The great thing about the flat belly diet isn't just the exceptional foods, weight loss, and smaller waist size, it is its popularity. This diet is incredibly popular worldwide, which means its resources are unsurpassed in quantity. No matter where you look online or in the media, even television morning shows are touting its incredible ability to deliver results in just over a month. If you would like to increase your seriousness, and exchange the terminology from "diet plan" to "lifestyle change" after the first month's success is evident, there are innumerable materials available to guide you successfully down the path of extended weight loss and healthy eating.

## *Online Resources*

There are a myriad of chat rooms, online forums and discussion groups that revolve around the flat belly diet. People are busy exchanging their results and ideas for continuing the highly successful dieting plan, and there is absolutely no reason why you should not get involved in the exchange.

You could learn healthy meal alternatives, as well as how others continued their success long after the first 32 days were over. Likewise, if you are struggling with any portion of the program, even if it is in the first couple days, seek support from others who are experiencing the same anxieties. These conversations usually result in supportive teamwork which allows all of the interested parties to commiserate for the duration of the program.

In the beginning of the diet, it will be incredibly important for you to let yourself be consumed by the process. This means having your meals at home, while preparing your meals for each day at the office, especially for the first four days of the program. In addition, you will be drinking a lot of Sassy water in those first few days, so be sure that you always have access to a bathroom. Ideally, you want to make yourself as comfortable as possible, so the challenges and obstacles are lessened immediately. The more roadblocks you put between you and the diet's constraints, which includes going to a sandwich shop with friends, instead of preparing a specific meal, the less likely you are to succeed.

The flat belly diet requires commitment, dedication and a serious attitude about the process. If by day three all you can talk about it how much the diet sucks, you will fail. Do your best to keep a positive attitude, and lean on your support system for help. This includes family, friends and online communities that can help you through the tougher days by providing encouragement. You will not want to surround yourself with people who have never dieted, and consider your attempt ridiculous. This is completely counterproductive to the process, and a way of introducing yourself to another opportunity for failure.

When you begin the diet, carry a notebook with you, complete with healthy food options that you can consume, so if you are forced into a lunchtime meeting that does not allow for your strict dieting constraints, you can reference the notebook for smart alternatives at a local restaurant. Be sure to write down what you eat every day, as keeping a food journal allows you to physically see the items you have consumed within a week. In fact, you should do this before you start the diet, even if for one week, so you can compare and contrast the two, which will provide you with an outstanding outline of where your food choices went wrong to begin with. The idea is not to make you feel bad about yourself, but to help you understand that making healthy lifestyle choices, especially where food is concerned, can make all of the difference in your weight and self-esteem.

If you are more of a self-starter, and prefer to lead by example, start a blog about your experience, and allow others to follow you along the journey. You can provide insight into how you are feeling after each day, or what times you feel more vulnerable to temptation and how you countered the sensation.

People love a great story, and want to feel like they are not the only ones who are struggling with their successes. Diets are not easy, which is why so many people give up on their New Year's resolutions so quickly. It is also why we're all not rail thin, and exercising for an hour each day. Keep in mind, with challenges come success, and keeping track of how this diet affects your life, whether through a public forum or a private journal, will help you come out on top, thinner, healthier and happier.

## Keeping the Weight Off

Diets, by their very definition, mean "absence of food". This derives a number of negative connotations, whether you are the one engaging in the diet, or are simply associated with someone who is. When people tell their friends that they are "on a diet" a number of emotions are stirred, including thoughts of inferiority, possibly by those who feel they could benefit from a diet as well, to a shaken confidence in what family meals are going to consist of for the duration of this period. It is safe to say, diets invite skepticism. Whether you are the practitioner or are simply bound to them socially, dieting is not an exciting topic.

With this knowledge, and the hard work and discipline it takes to lose the weight, the very last thing you are going to want to experience is for it all to come back! The very yo-yo diet you have tried all too many times before has hopefully been displaced by the incredible dieting solution that is the Flat Belly Diet. Making this diet a part of your life, and gaining healthy eating alternatives from its use, should help you maintain your optimal weight. However, it is important for any dieter to note that food sources are not the only contributors to weight gain. Stress, lack of sleep, and assuming a sedentary lifestyle will each send your weight reeling, making it twice as hard to resume your Flat Belly appearance.

# Stress

Obstinate belly fat is not only a menace to any dieter's bottom line, and almost always the focal point of results, but its overall stubbornness can be attributed to stress levels. Whether your stress levels are heightened through your work or home life, or are rooted chemically, emotionally or physically, it will cause fat accumulation.

When stress becomes a factor in anyone's life, their cortisol levels are raised. Usually, if someone is in a stressful situation, they would use that feeling or rise in adrenaline to motivate themselves into movement. For instance, if someone threatens you, invoking a stressful assertion, fight or flight kicks in and you are able to respond to those cortisol levels through movement. The problem is, people are surrounded by stressful situations at home, work and socially, where they are unable to remove themselves from the environment and relieve the stress. If your boss yells at you, you cannot simply get up and run a mile the moment it happens. If your home life is full of strife, chances are you are stuck to deal with it, instead of being able to kick box at the drop of a hat. The problem is, when stress mounts, it mounts in your abdomen, and invites stubborn fat to join it. This is the very reason that people cannot seem to lose their belly fat, no matter what type of diet they are pursuing.

## Relieving Stress

In addition to maintaining a healthy, flat belly diet approach, it is important to provide yourself with stress relief solutions. This is absolutely no time to be naïve: Everyone has stress. Yours just may manifest differently from someone else's, but it does not make it any less harmful. There are a few ways to help relieve stress, without joining a gym.

## Get Some Sleep

Adults require seven to eight hours of sleep each night. However, most adults know that is simply an insane request. Children, busy lives, careers, travel and the fact that there are only twenty four hours available in each day can hinder anyone from spending a third of it in bed. Adjust your schedule as much as you can to get an optimum amount of sleep. If you are only able to get six hours of sleep each night, make them the best six hours you can. This means removing any technological items from your bedroom, including laptops, tablets, cell phones, and televisions. Use your bedroom solely for the purpose of sleeping, so your body knows once you enter that room, it is time to relax completely. In addition, try to maintain a steady schedule for that room's use. Do not work in your bedroom, or use it as a social gathering place for your family to vent their needs. Your bedroom should be your safe haven, and if it is possible to insure that you use it from midnight to six am each day, than do so. The body loves a schedule; especially one that allows it to rest comfortably.

## Relax, Breathe & Meditate

Meditation is sometimes perceived as a lengthy exercise that can only be accomplished with the proper clothing, exercise mat, candles and confusing music. Nothing could be further from the truth. Meditation is practiced by sitting quietly and comfortably, with your eyes closed and body still, in an attempt to clear the mind of any cluttered anxiety or oppressive thoughts that are weighing you down. Whether you prefer to do this alone, in a class, at your desk, or in your bedroom, the principle is the same: relieve stress.

## Exercise

To be clear, this diet does not require a workout regimen to be successful. The program simply suggests that you start moving around a lot more than you have in the past, in an effort to stimulate weight loss. However, if your stress levels are keeping you from completely experiencing this diet and its benefits, it may be time to work an exercise class into your week.

Instead of overwhelming yourself with promises of going to the gym each day, which almost any busy person can tell you is practically impossible, consider taking a single workout class, once a week.

Spinning, aerobics, yoga or even a dance class are great ways to work off stress, without taking more than an hour out of your existing workload. Consider joining a running club, or asking friends to meet you for a "Boot camp" style workout once a week. Exercise is a great outlet for stress, so don't be afraid to use it.

# Closing Notes

## Be Yourself

People diet for a number of reasons, but most of those can be attributed to weight loss. But why? Are you dieting because YOU want to? Or because everyone around you is dieting? Maintaining a healthy weight is incredibly important to your health, so whatever your catalyst for delving into the flat belly diet should be applauded. However, your body may not work like your best friend's body does. You may not see the same results, or you may benefit from them quicker than someone else. The important thing to remember is that you are officially taking control of your health, and your appearance and self-esteem will begin to reap the rewards in no time. While you are getting there, maintain your own goals, food schedule, exercise plan and outlook. This is your diet, and although sharing it with others to provide advice or motivation is priceless, it is also important that you are happy with the process. A successful flat belly diet plan will provide you with confidence so embrace it and nurture it!

Once you have developed the new you, keep up with your new look and energy by purchasing a new outfit, or welcoming new challenges into your life in the form of activities with your family or friends. Discovering things you like to do will help you keep your new, healthier body intact, so start thinking about your life in the form of doing more. Do you like to hike, ride bikes, rock climb? Perhaps swimming and sunbathing are more your speed? Make a list of things you like to do, and refer to it often. In addition, make a list of all the things you like about the new you, and add to it every chance you get. Your soaring self-esteem will be on full display, allowing you to be more comfortable in your own skin. That is precisely what all dieters want, and the Flat Belly Diet delivers.

# The End

# RECOMMENDED READS

## Eat to Live: The Amazing Nutrient-Rich Program for Fast and Sustained Weight Loss
By Joel Fuhrman

## Wheat Belly: Lose the Wheat, Lose the Weight, and Find Your Path Back To Health
By William Davis MD

## The 5:2 Diet Book:
Feast for 5 Days a Week and Fast for 2 to Lose Weight, Boost Your Brain and Transform Your Health
By Kate Harrison

## The Virgin Diet:
Drop 7 Foods, Lose 7 Pounds, Just 7 Days
By JJ Virgin

# About the Author

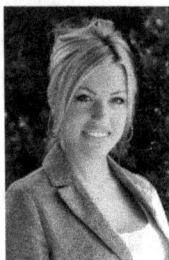

Mackenzie Jagger was born and raised in Baltimore, Maryland. Currently an event planner that recently turned 30 enjoys reading and writing about diet and fitness related subjects. She says her boyfriend is a bodybuilder and fitness "nut" and inspires her to be her best. She also loves to sing and dance.

Mackenzie Jagger's Author Page

https://www.amazon.com/author/mackenziejagger

Mackenzie Jagger's Website

http://TheFlatBellySolution.org

No part of this publication may be copied, reproduced in any format, by any means, electronic or otherwise, without prior consent from the copyright owner and publisher of this book.

**DISCLAIMER:** THIS INFORMATION IS NOT PRESENTED BY A MEDICAL PRACTITIONER AND IS FOR EDUCATIONAL AND INFORMATIONAL PURPOSES ONLY. THE CONTENT IS NOT INTENDED TO BE A SUBSTITUTE FOR PROFESSIONAL MEDICAL ADVICE, DIAGNOSIS, OR TREATMENT. ALWAYS SEEK THE ADVICE OF YOUR PHYSICIAN OR OTHER QUALIFIED HEALTH CARE PROVIDER WITH ANY QUESTIONS YOU MAY HAVE REGARDING A MEDICAL CONDITION. NEVER DISREGARD PROFESSIONAL MEDICAL ADVICE OR DELAY IN SEEKING IT BECAUSE OF SOMETHING YOU HAVE READ.

www.ingramcontent.com/pod-product-compliance
Lightning Source LLC
Chambersburg PA
CBHW050552280326
41933CB00011B/1817